Your Guide to

Total Knee Replacement

Fairview Health Services

Minneapolis, Minnesota

Published by Fairview Press, 2450 Riverside Avenue, Minneapolis, Minnesota 55454. Fairview Press is a division of Fairview Health Services, a community-focused health system affiliated with the University of Minnesota and providing a complete range of services, from the prevention of illness and injury to care for the most complex medical conditions.

Library of Congress Cataloging-in-Publication Data
Your guide to total knee replacement / Fairview Health Services.
    p. cm.
  Includes bibliographical references.
  ISBN-13: 978-1-57749-165-1 (pbk. : alk. paper)
  ISBN-10: 1-57749-165-3 (pbk. : alk. paper)
  1. Total knee replacement--Popular works. I. Fairview Health Services. II. Title: Total knee replacement.
  RD561.Y68 2007
  617.5'820592--dc22

                                        2006021473

First Printing: January 2007
Printed in the United States of America
11 10 09 08 07   6 5 4 3 2 1

Edited by Lee Engfer
Illustrations by Laurie Ingram

Medical Disclaimer
This publication is designed to provide accurate and authoritative information in regard to the subject matter covered. It is sold with the understanding that the publisher is not engaged in the provision or practice of medical, nursing, or professional health care advice or services in any jurisdiction. If medical advice or other professional assistance is required, the services of a qualified and competent professional should be sought. Fairview Press is not responsible or liable, directly or indirectly, for any form of damages whatsoever resulting from the use (or misuse) of information contained in or implied by these documents.

Customized editions of this publication (imprinted with your institution's name, contact information, etc.) are also available. Contact Fairview Press at 612-672-4774 for pricing.

Contents

Introduction

Total knee replacement is surgery to replace a painful knee joint. The surgery can help you get back to doing the things you want to do.

As you get ready for surgery you may have a lot of questions. Many people find it helpful to learn as much as they can about total knee replacement. This book lets you know what to expect before, during and after surgery.

Fairview Health Services developed this book as a learning tool. Our goal is to give you basic facts about total knee replacement and help you plan for your surgery, hospital stay and recovery. This book also offers tips for living with your new knee. It will help you understand the goals you'll work toward and the guidelines for knee safety.

Please take some time to read the whole book before your surgery. You don't have to read it all at once—go at your own pace. If you have questions, ask your doctor or nurse.

Your health care team

Your health care team will work together during your surgery, hospital stay and recovery. You and your family are the most important members of your health care team. You will help your recovery by taking an active role in your care.

Along with your doctor and surgeon, members of your health care team include:

- **Nurses.** A team of nurses and support staff will help with your care plan before and after surgery. They talk with other care providers to make sure all parts of your care work together. They help with your daily activities (including exercises and walking), treatments, personal care, pain relief and planning for when you leave the hospital.

- **Physical therapists.** These team members are trained to help you move safely with your new knee. They will work with you to strengthen your muscles before and after surgery. Physical therapists will develop an exercise program for you and show you how to do the movements. They will also show you how to use a walker or crutches.

- **Occupational therapists.** These therapists will teach you how to dress, manage personal care and do household tasks safely with your new knee. They will show you how to use equipment you may need to perform these tasks.

Tip
_____

Don't forget: You are the most important member of your health care team.

- **Social workers and care coordinators.** These team members help you and your family plan for when you leave the hospital. They can tell you about helpful resources and talk with you about your insurance, or health plan.

Please tell you care team if you need a language interpreter or are deaf or hard of hearing. You have the right to a trained medical interpreter who will help you talk with doctors and nurses.

You might also want to ask if spiritual support is available at your hospital. Most hospitals have chaplains who support a range of faith traditions. Or you may contact your own faith community for support.

What Is Knee Replacement?

Your knees allow you to walk, climb stairs and bend. The knee joint is the place where bones of the upper and lower legs connect. It is where motion occurs.

The knees are the most complex joints in the body. Not only do they bend and straighten, but they also twist and turn. You use your knees for a wide range of movements.

A painful knee can make it harder to enjoy an active life. A knee that is damaged or worn down can't take the daily demands it once did.

Total knee replacement is surgery to remove the parts of the knee that are damaged and replace them with new parts. This can ease your pain and get you moving again. Knee replacement is one of the most common and successful surgeries.

Understanding your knee

The knee is a large, complex joint. It is made up of three bones held together by tough bands of tissue called ligaments. The thighbone (femur) makes up the top part of the joint. It meets the shinbone (tibia) at the lower part of the knee joint. In front of these bones is the kneecap (patella). This is the bone you feel when you touch your knee. The kneecap is like a round shield that protects the joint. It glides in a groove on the end of the thighbone whenever you bend or straighten your leg.

A normal, healthy knee

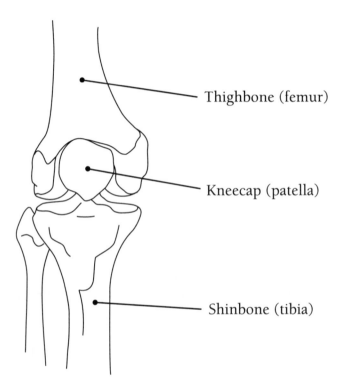

Thighbone (femur)

Kneecap (patella)

Shinbone (tibia)

The thighbone and shinbone are separated by cartilage, a smooth, tough tissue that keeps the bones from rubbing together. (You've probably seen cartilage on the end of a chicken drumstick.) The cartilage acts as a cushion or padding. It allows the two bones to move together so you can bend your knee.

Muscles and ligaments surround the knee joint and keep it stable as it moves. The main muscles of the knee include the quadriceps, in the front of the knee, and the hamstrings, in the back of the knee. Four main ligaments connect the thighbone to the shinbone.

A painful knee

If your knee is hurt or worn down, the joint does not move smoothly. Movement becomes painful. You may have trouble putting weight on that leg. You might limp and find it hard to walk. Your knee may be stiff or swollen, making it hard to bend and straighten. A painful knee can keep you from doing the things you enjoy.

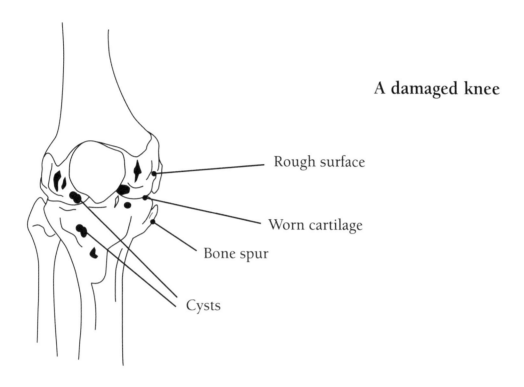

A damaged knee

Rough surface

Worn cartilage

Bone spur

Cysts

What can go wrong

The most common reason for knee replacement is a disease called osteoarthritis (AHS-tee-oh-arth-RY-tuss). The cartilage wears away from the bones, causing the joint to lose its cushion. The surface of the bones becomes rough. The rough edges of the bones may rub against each other, causing pain. The knee may become swollen.

As the pain gets worse, you may try to stop using your knee. This causes the muscles around the joint to weaken. People with arthritis in the knee have trouble walking, climbing stairs and getting in and out of a chair. The knee may bend less than usual and it will not straighten all the way.

Sometimes osteoarthritis occurs because of:

- A broken bone in the knee

- Torn cartilage or ligaments in the knee joint

- Past injuries that create extra wear and tear on the joint

- Rheumatoid (ROOM-uh-toyd) arthritis, a disease that causes stiffness, swelling and pain in the joints

Getting a new knee

In total knee replacement surgery, doctors remove damaged cartilage from your thighbone, shinbone and kneecap. They replace these with new parts made of metal and strong plastic.

Surgery usually lasts about two hours. A 4- to 6-inch cut (incision) is made to gain access to the knee joint. After removing the diseased bone and cartilage, doctors prepare the remaining bone for the implant (the new knee). The upper part of the implant fits into your thighbone, and the lower part fits into your shinbone. The new kneecap fits over the front of the implant.

The doctor may wedge the pieces tightly into place or fix them to the bones with special cement. Your doctor will decide which method is best for you.

If you have pain in both knees, the surgeon may suggest having both knees replaced at the same time (called bilateral knee replacement). In this case, you only have to have surgery once instead of twice. If you and your doctor agree that this is the best option, you may need to spend some time in a care facility after your surgery.

Minimally invasive surgery

A new technique in knee replacement is known as "minimally invasive surgery." Basically, it's the same operation as traditional knee replacement, but it's done through smaller incisions (cuts in the skin). The artificial parts are the same in both operations.

In a traditional knee replacement, the surgeon makes a 4- to 6-inch cut along the side of the knee. The surgeon has to cut through muscles and several ligaments to get to the knee joint. In the newer technique, the surgeon makes one cut of 3 to 6 inches, or two cuts of 1 to 3 inches each. With the smaller incision, the surgeon can operate between muscles and ligaments instead of cutting through them.

Doctors who have performed this technique say it can result in less pain and a faster recovery time. For a traditional knee replacement, the patient is in the hospital for two to four days. The person uses crutches or a walker for five to six weeks. With minimally invasive surgery, the hospital stay is as little as one day. People feel less soreness and are able to get up and move around sooner. They use crutches for just about a week.

Minimally invasive surgery is a developing and evolving field. If you will be having this kind of surgery, please ask your surgeon which parts of this book apply to you.

Partial Knee Replacement

Partial (unicompartmental) knee replacement may be an option for people who have damage in just one section of the knee joint. The knee still has some healthy cartilage. In a partial knee replacement, the surgeon replaces only the most damaged area of the joint with new parts.

In this surgery, the cut (incision) is smaller than the one needed for total knee replacement. The hospital stay is shorter, and your knee may heal more quickly. For most people with arthritis and other knee problems, however, there is too much damage for a partial replacement.

The artificial knee

The artificial joint, or implant, is called a prosthesis (PRAHSS-thee-sis). It has three parts:

*   The upper part (femoral component) replaces the end of the thighbone. This part is made of titanium, stainless steel or another long-lasting metal.

*   The lower part (tibial component) fits into the end of the shinbone. It is made of metal and sturdy plastic.

*   The kneecap part (patellar component) replaces all or part of the kneecap. It fits over the front of the other two parts.

These parts fit together to create a new knee with smooth surfaces. The new parts touch and glide against each other in a natural, comfortable motion. This allows your knee to bend and straighten.

A new knee joint (prosthesis)

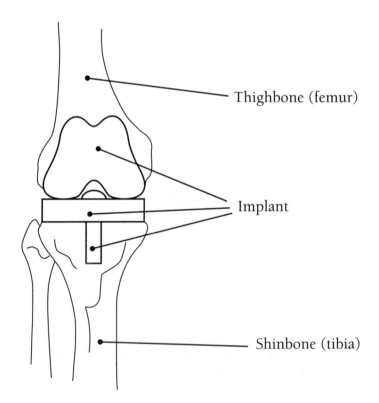

Thighbone (femur)

Implant

Shinbone (tibia)

What to expect from surgery

The goal of knee replacement surgery is to reduce pain and stiffness. For most people, the surgery does just that. Long-term studies have shown pain relief in 90 to 95 percent of people who have this surgery.

After the pain from the surgery goes away, you will likely notice that your arthritis pain is gone, too. Most people have no ongoing pain, or they have a small amount that they control with over-the-counter medicine. People often feel less stiffness as well.

After healing, you'll be able to get back to many of the things you normally do, such as walking, biking, golfing, dancing and swimming. For more than nine out of 10 people, their new knee lasts 10 years or more.

Questions to Ask Your Doctor

Before surgery, you will feel more prepared if you talk with your health care team and review this book. Write down any other questions you have so you don't forget to ask them. Be sure to ask:

- What are the short-term and long-term risks of this surgery?

- What can I do to get ready for surgery?

- Can I take my medicines before surgery?

- How long will it take for me to recover?

- When can I start driving again?

- How long will I walk with a walker, cane or crutches?

- Can I ever kneel on my new knee?

- When can I go back to work?

- What kind of help do you think I'll need in the first couples weeks after surgery?

The risks of surgery

Like any major surgery, knee replacement brings certain risks. Major problems, while uncommon, can be treated.

When a new knee fails, it is often due to infection or to loosening slowly over time (where the metal or cement meets the bone). Other common risks are:

- Blood clots in the leg or lung

- Problems urinating (passing water when using the toilet)

- Nerve damage

- Some knee pain

- Stiffness

Some of these problems happen soon after surgery. Others may not show up until years later.

Most problems can be prevented. Your health care team will show you how to move safely with your new knee and reduce the risk of problems. (See "Preventing complications," page 42.)

Planning Ahead for Your Recovery

After knee surgery, it may be several months before you can do all the things you are used to doing. You can make this time easier by planning ahead.

The time to make plans for leaving the hospital is *before* you go in for surgery. The more ready you are, the more smoothly things will go at the hospital and at home. This chapter offers tips to make recovery easier.

Make a recovery plan

Most people stay in the hospital for three nights after surgery. If you're having both knees replaced, the hospital stay will be four or five nights. Your health care team will help you form a plan for leaving the hospital (called a discharge plan). This plan is based on your needs, your progress in using your new knee and your insurance coverage.

During your hospital stay you will work toward a number of goals, such as getting in and out of bed safely and walking with your walker, crutches or cane. Your health care team will let you know if you can go straight home from the hospital or if you will need extra help.

Home

You can go home after leaving the hospital if you can:

- Get in and out of bed and a chair by yourself or with a little help from a caregiver

- Walk with your walker, crutches or cane

- Walk the distance from your bedroom to your bathroom and kitchen

- Safely get on and off the toilet by yourself or with a little help

- Go up and down the stairs safely

At home you will need help from family and friends for several weeks. You may need help with dressing, personal care and household tasks.

Your energy level will be lower than usual. Over time you will need less help. If you are going right home after surgery, ask a family member, friend or neighbor to stay close by for the first few days to a week. If you live alone or are alone during the day, plan for someone to stay with you for at least the first few days to a week. Decide who will take you home from the hospital and drive you to doctor visits.

Home with home health services

If you can go home but will need more help, you may qualify for home health services. In this case, nurses, home health aides or physical or occupational therapists will visit you at home. They can help you with walking, strengthening exercises, daily activities and safety issues. They will also keep track of your overall health.

Your care team will let you know if you need these services. Talk with a social worker or care coordinator at the hospital to see if your insurance plan covers home health visits.

Tip

_____

Arrange for a friend or family member to stay with you for the first week after surgery.

If you already use home health services, bring the agency's name and phone number to the hospital. Your social worker or care coordinator can help increase the amount of care you will receive at home. If you have not used home health services in the past, ask your care coordinator to help you find a home health agency.

Skilled nursing facility

Some people need more services than they can get at home. If this is true for you, you may need to spend a week or longer in a skilled nursing facility. (This is sometimes called an extended care facility, transitional care unit or "step-down" care facility.)

For example, if you're having both knees replaced, you will likely need to spend some time at a care facility. Caregivers there will attend to your medical needs until you can safely return home. You will also get physical therapy every day. Therapy will help you build your strength and self-care skills. The care team will work with you and your family so you can go home as quickly as possible.

Your social worker or care coordinator can help you find a place that offers the short-term care you need. Try to find three facilities where you would feel comfortable. Call your insurance company to find out if these places are covered under your plan.

Understand your health insurance coverage

Health care benefits differ from one plan to another, and benefits often change. Before you have surgery, be sure you know what your insurance plan covers. Call your health plan or look at your policy book. Find out exactly what is and is not covered after surgery. Ask about home health care, a skilled nursing facility and medical equipment.

Make a living will

A health care directive (also called an advance directive or living will) lets you decide what medical care you would want if you became unable to communicate. It tells your family about your wishes for treatment, such as whether you would want to be on a life-support machine.

Tip

Know what your insurance plan will pay for. Ask about home health care, a skilled nursing facility and medical equipment.

A health care directive is useful for all adults, even those who are not facing major surgery. It is a written, legal document. Your family and medical team can turn to the directive if you become unable to make your own health care decisions.

Bring a copy of your health care directive to the hospital. It will be part of your files. If you don't have a health care directive, you may wish to ask for the form you need to make a living will.

Plan for less activity

Your schedule will need to change after surgery, as you will not be able to do as much. Your movements and energy level will be limited. Let people know you will be "out of action" for a while. If you work, arrange for time off for the surgery and recovery. Talk to your health care team about how long you will need to be away from work.

Prepare your home

Tip

Set up a recovery station— the place where you will spend the most time after surgery. Keep the things you will use most within easy reach.

Another important step is to make your home safe and easy for you to get around. After surgery, you won't be able to kneel down, stoop or use a low toilet or furniture.

These limits can make it hard to do things you take for granted. Cooking and cleaning bring new challenges. Even something as simple as watching TV requires thought about where you keep the remote and whether you have to bend down to use a VCR or DVD player.

Before surgery, make your home as accessible as possible. Follow the tips on page 14 to 15 ("Getting your home ready for your return"). Set up a "recovery station" where you will spend most of your time. In this handy spot, keep the things you use most—the TV remote control, phone, medicine, books, magazines, reading glasses, tissues, waste basket, a pitcher of water and a glass for drinking.

Stock up on basic groceries and meals that are quick and easy to make. It's a good idea to prepare some meals in advance and freeze them. Frozen casseroles and soups can be reheated and served easily.

Talk to a physical or occupational therapist about equipment you may need to install in your home. You may rent or buy items that make it easier for you to use the bathtub, toilet and other areas. For a list of items that can help, see chapter 5.

If You Live Alone

Before you go to the hospital, ask your health care team how to set up your home to make your tasks easier. You will need someone to stay with you for the first few days to a week. After that, think about the tasks you will need help with. Ask family and friends for help with the things you can't do on your own.

Here are some things to think about if you live alone.

- Find someone to help care for your pet while you're in the hospital.

- Ask a neighbor to do your outdoor work, such as lawn mowing or shoveling, while you are healing.

- Make plans to have someone drive you to the grocery store, religious services, family events and doctor and therapy visits. Keep a list of people who are willing to take turns helping out.

- If you don't have many people to help you, talk with your social worker or care coordinator. He or she can put you in touch with resources in your area.

Getting Your Home Ready for Your Return

General

- Leave your home clean and tidy so you won't have to clean it when you return.

- Keep a phone near your bed and main living area. Post emergency numbers on or near the phones. When you are home alone, carry a cordless or mobile phone.

- Move items that you use often to arm level, so you don't have to reach up or bend down.

- Remove throw rugs. Tape down the edges of large area rugs.

- Remove clutter from hallways and other pathways. Keep walkways free of furniture as well as electrical and phone cords.

- If you have stairs in your home, make sure there is a handrail. Check railings to be sure they are not wobbly. If you are adding a new handrail, it should extend a few inches past the end of the staircase.

- Be sure you have enough light indoors, outdoors and in stairways. Put night-lights in dark hallways.

- Ask your mail and newspaper carriers to deliver to your door. If possible, have packages and newspapers placed on a bench, rather than on the floor.

Bedroom

- Use a regular bed with a box spring and mattress. If your bed is upstairs, think about moving it to the main floor for the weeks of recovery.

- Leave extra space around your bed. This gives you room to get in and out while using crutches, a walker or a cane.

- Keep a flashlight next to your bed. Or use night-lights for nighttime trips to the bathroom.

Getting Your Home Ready for Your Return

Bathroom

- Install a raised toilet seat. (See page 58.)

- Use a rubber mat or put nonskid tape strips in the bathtub or shower stall. This helps prevent falls.

- If your bathroom is not on the main floor where you're sleeping, look into getting a commode or portable toilet. (See page 58.)

- Put grab bars in the bathtub or shower. You may also need grab bars by the toilet.

- Install a hand-held showerhead to make bathing easier. (See page 59.)

- Liquid soap may be easier to use than bar soap, which can slip away.

Kitchen

- Use a cart to move heavy or hot items.

- Place utensils where you can reach them without bending or stretching.

- It may be hard to use the dishwasher. Instead, use a dish drainer in the sink or on the counter.

- Plan to use the microwave for cooking. If you want to use the stove, leave saucepans on the stove or at stovetop height.

Recovery plan timeline

It will take several weeks to plan your recovery and get ready for surgery. While everyone's needs are different, these are the basic steps you will need to take.

6 weeks before surgery

☐ Arrange for the help you will need during your recovery. If you will be at home, ask someone to stay with you for the first few days to a week. Make sure you have people to drive you to buy groceries, go to the doctor, etc.

☐ Schedule your pre-surgery exam anytime within 30 days of your surgery date.

☐ Call your insurance company to review your coverage for when you are in the hospital and when you leave.

☐ Go to the dentist, if you haven't gone within the last year.

☐ Eat a well-balanced, healthy diet.

☐ Start doing your strengthening exercises. (See page 20.)

☐ Write down any questions you have about your hospital stay and recovery. You can ask these at your pre-surgery exam. For questions about your surgery, call the surgeon's office.

3 weeks before surgery

☐ Get your home ready for your recovery. Make some meals that you can freeze and reheat later. Stock up on basic foods and easy-to-make meals.

☐ Have your pre-surgery exam and blood tests, if you haven't already. You need to do this within 30 days of your surgery.

☐ If you live alone and have a pet, arrange for someone to take care of the pet while you're in the hospital.

☐ Stop mail and newspaper delivery, unless someone will bring them in for you.

☐ Keep doing your strengthening exercises.

Tip
_____

Schedule your pre-surgery exam several weeks in advance.

1 week before surgery

- ☐ Talk to your doctor about the medicines you take. Find out which ones you need to stop taking.

- ☐ Stop taking aspirin, ibuprofen and other anti-inflammatory drugs (such as Aleve). Tylenol is okay.

- ☐ Continue doing your strengthening exercises.

- ☐ Learn the breathing exercises you'll do after surgery. (See page 25.) Practice them every day.

1 day before surgery

- ☐ Pack the items you will bring to the hospital.

- ☐ Follow the rules your health care team gave you about diet and bathing.

- ☐ Make sure you have a ride to and from the hospital.

Tip
_____

Don't forget to arrange for a ride to and from the hospital.

Getting Ready for Surgery

Before you have major surgery, you want to be in the best shape you can be. This means you should be in good health. If you have any sign of illness, severe heart or lung disease or other problems, your surgery may have to be postponed.

You will want to strengthen your upper-body and leg muscles before surgery. You should also learn your breathing exercises. All of this will help with your recovery.

Staying healthy

The better your overall health is, the less likely you are to have problems during or after surgery. To stay in good health:

- **Eat a healthy diet.** Good nutrition can help you heal and lower the chance of infection. A healthy diet includes plenty of fruits and vegetables and is low in fat and sugar. If you have questions or concerns about your diet, talk to a nurse or dietician.

- **Stop smoking.** If you quit smoking, even the week before surgery, it will lower your risks from surgery. You are not allowed to smoke in the hospital. If you need help quitting, tell your care team.

Tip
_____

*See your dentist six weeks
before surgery. If your gums
or teeth get infected, you
are more likely to get an
infection in the knee.*

- **Stay active.** Exercise improves your heart and lungs and boosts your immune system. But staying active when your knee hurts can be tough. Try swimming and water exercises. These give you exercise without putting stress on your knees.

- **Take care of your teeth.** If you have not had a dental checkup within the last year, see your dentist at least six weeks before surgery. When teeth or gums become infected, bacteria (germs) can travel to the new knee joint. If the tissue around your new knee gets infected, you may need more surgery. It's best to have dental work done well before your knee is replaced.

Strengthening exercises

You may have become less active because of the pain and stiffness in your knee. When muscles are not used, they become weak. After you have your knee replaced, the joint problem will be fixed, but your muscles may still be weak. To make them stronger, you will follow a regular exercise program.

Start doing your exercises before your surgery. This way, it will be easier to do them after surgery. Getting stronger now will also speed your recovery.

Tip
_____

*Start your exercises now.
This will help you heal
faster after surgery.*

You will strengthen the muscles in your legs and buttocks. These will support your new knee joint. It's also a good idea to strengthen your upper-body muscles. These will help you pull yourself up, sit up and push yourself around in bed. Strong arms also help you use crutches or a walker.

Practice the following exercises before your surgery. Most of these exercises are done lying down. You can do them in bed if you like. **Do not hold your breath while you exercise.**

Repeat each exercise 10 times or until your muscle feels tired. You are the best judge of how much you can do each day. If you feel pain, stop doing that exercise.

Ankle pumps and circles

For pumps, slowly flex your foot toward you, then away from you. For circles, move your foot around in circles, first in one direction, then the other.

Thigh squeezes

Lying flat, press the back of your knee into the bed. At the same time, tighten your thigh. Hold for 5 seconds. Switch legs.

Buttocks squeezes

Tighten your buttocks muscles by squeezing them together. Hold for 5 seconds.

Hamstring sets

Slightly bend the knee on the side of your bad leg. Tighten the muscle at the back of your thigh (hamstring) by pressing your heel into the bed. Hold for 5 seconds.

Heel slides

Lying flat, slide your heel toward your buttocks, bending your knee. Keep your heel on the bed and your kneecap pointed to the ceiling. Repeat with other heel.

Lying kicks

Lie on your back. Place a rolled-up blanket under the knee of your sore leg. Straighten your knee, keeping the back of your thigh on the blanket the whole time. Hold for 5 seconds.

Straight leg raises

Lie flat on your back. With your knee straight, tighten your thigh muscle. As your thigh muscle tightens, lift your leg several inches off the bed. Keep your leg straight. Hold for 5 seconds, then slowly lower your leg.

Bed sit-ups

Lie flat on your back. Come up on both elbows, then up on both hands. With your arms straight out behind you, come to a sitting position. Now reverse: lower yourself onto your elbows, then flat on your back.

Sitting kicks

Sit in a sturdy chair. Straighten the knee of one leg as much as you can. Hold your leg up for 5 seconds. Switch legs.

Knee bends

Sit on a chair. Pull your leg back toward the chair as much as you can. You will feel the stretch in your knee. Return to the starting position and relax. To increase the stretch, scoot forward on the chair.

Chair push-ups

Sit in a sturdy chair with arms, or in a wheelchair with the wheels locked. Hold the chair arms. Push down on the chair arms and straighten your elbows. Push yourself up off the chair as much as you can, then slowly lower yourself back down.

Breathing exercises

After surgery, you will be asked to do breathing exercises. These help prevent pneumonia and other lung problems. The exercises include deep breathing and coughing. It's a good idea to learn these exercises before surgery. Practice them every day for at least a week before you go in the hospital.

Deep breathing

Deep breathing helps fill your lungs completely. When you are doing it right, deep breathing uses your stomach muscles as well as your chest muscles.

1. Breathe in through your nose as deeply as you can. Hold for several seconds. Your stomach should go out as you breathe in.

2. Let your breath out through your mouth, slowly, so that all the breath goes out. Purse your lips as you breathe out, as if you were blowing out a candle. Your stomach should go in as you breathe out.

Breathe out for twice as long as you breathe in. Repeat 10 times.

Coughing

Coughing helps keep your lungs clear. Follow these steps.

1. Take a slow, deep breath. Breathe in through your nose. Focus on fully expanding your chest and back.

2. Breathe out through your mouth. Feel your chest sink downward and inward.

3. Take another breath in the same way.

4. Take a third breath. This time, hold your breath for a moment and then cough hard. As you cough, focus on forcing all the air out of your chest.

Repeat this exercise two more times.

Tip

_____

If you practice your breathing exercises before surgery, they will be easier to do afterward—and you will be less likely to have lung problems.

Pre-surgery exam

Tip

Write down the name and dose of every medicine, herb and vitamin you take. Bring this list to your health exam.

You will see your doctor for a checkup within 30 days of your surgery. At this time you may have several tests, including blood tests. These tests give a good picture of your overall health.

During this exam, it's important to tell your doctor about all your medicines. Bring a written list of your medicines and the amounts you normally take. Also bring a list of past surgeries and hospital stays.

One week before surgery, you will need to stop taking aspirin and anti-inflammatory medicines. (These are drugs that reduce fever and swelling. They include Advil, Motrin, Aleve, Naprosyn, Feldene, Relafen, DayPro and others.) If you take these medicines every day for pain, ask your doctor how you can relieve pain during the week before surgery.

Your doctor will tell you if you need to stop any other medicines before surgery. Make sure you know:

- When to stop taking your medicines

- When to stop taking vitamins and herbal products (such as gingko, St. John's wort, garlic or echinacea)

- Which medicines you should take the morning of surgery, and how to take them (including diabetes medicines)

If you aren't sure if the drugs you take should be stopped, ask your doctor.

The day before surgery

- **Diet.** It's important to have an empty stomach before surgery. This will make the surgery as safe as possible. Your surgeon will tell you when to stop eating and drinking. **If you don't follow his or her orders, your surgery could be changed to another date.**

- **Bathing.** You will be told when and how to bathe before surgery. You will use anti-bacterial soap, such as Dial, or the special soap you get from your doctor. This soap helps kill germs and prevent infection.

- **Changes in health.** Call your doctor if there is any change in your health. Examples include a sore throat, runny nose, cough, fever, dental problems, urinating problems or skin problems, such as a rash, scrape or cut. These may mean that your surgery has to be postponed.

- **Other tips.** Do not smoke, drink alcohol or take over-the-counter medicine (unless your surgeon tells you to) for 24 hours before surgery.

If you have any questions about your surgery or how to get ready, call your surgeon's office.

Tip

Be sure to follow the rules for eating and drinking before surgery. If you have any questions, call your surgeon's office.

Your Hospital Stay

Your care team will tell you what to expect at the hospital.

Before surgery

After checking in at the hospital, you will be asked to sign one or more consent forms. These forms state that you know the risks and benefits of surgery. When you sign the forms, you give your care team permission to do the surgery. Do not sign them unless you understand what will happen during and after your surgery.

Next you will go to the pre-surgery area, where you will be "prepped" (prepared) for surgery. Friends and family can stay with you there. When you're in surgery, they will be in the waiting area.

Anesthesia

An anesthesia provider will talk with you about what kind of anesthesia (medicine) will be used. This medicine will keep you comfortable during surgery. The provider will check your health status and answer any questions you have about the medicine.

You will have either general or regional anesthesia. The choice depends on the type of surgery you're having, your health history and your current health.

With **general anesthesia** you are asleep during surgery. You may receive the medicine through your IV tube or breathe it in through your nose. During surgery, a breathing tube helps you breathe while you are asleep. Afterward, you may feel some minor side effects, such as a sore throat, headache, hoarse voice, feeling sick to your stomach and feeling sleepy.

Regional anesthesia will make you lose all feeling from your lower back to your toes. You may receive this medicine through a shot in your lower back (called spinal anesthesia). It does not put you to sleep, but you may remember very little about the surgery. This is due to other medicines you may receive through your IV line. The most common side effects are small headaches that last for a few days and trouble passing urine when using the toilet.

After surgery

Surgery takes from one to four hours. With the "prep" time and wake-up time, you'll be in the operating room and recovery room for several hours.

It could take one to three hours for your anesthesia to wear off. In the recovery room, nurses will check your blood pressure, pulse and breathing. They will help you with any side effects from the anesthesia.

When you wake up:

- You may have an oxygen mask.

- You might have blurred vision and a dry mouth.

- You may feel sick to your stomach. If you vomit (throw up) or feel sick, you may be given medicine to help you feel better.

- You may be confused, drowsy and dizzy. Don't try to get up alone—you may be weaker than you think. Your nurse will help you when you first try to walk.

- You may feel some pain. Your nurse will make you as comfortable as possible. He or she will ask you to rate your pain using a pain scale. This tells your care team how much pain medicine to give you. If you had spinal anesthesia, you might not feel any pain right after surgery.

- A large bandage will cover the surgical area to keep it clean.

- You may have tubes that drain fluid from the surgical wound. (This is called an incision drain.) The fluid goes into a special container. Your care team will keep track of the amount of fluid that comes out.

- You'll receive fluids and medicines through an IV line in your arm.

- You may have a tube (catheter) in your bladder to remove urine.

When you are fully awake, you will be moved to your hospital room. Your family and friends can visit you there. You might have a room to yourself, or you may share a room with another patient.

Dealing with pain

As your body heals, you might feel a stabbing, pinching or aching pain. Treating pain is an important part of your care.

Tell your health care team about any pain you feel. Remember, all pain is real. You have the right to have it treated.

Your pain can be affected by how you feel about other things in your life. For example, worries about your job, money or family can cause stress and make your pain worse. Share your worries with your health care team. They can help you deal with the issues that add to your stress and pain.

Pain scale

Everyone feels pain in a different way. You may be asked to rate your pain using a pain scale. This will help your care team know how much pain you feel.

Tell your health care team:

- Where you feel pain and how much pain you have

- What makes your pain better or worse

- Which pain medicines have worked for you in the past

There are many ways to relieve pain. Your care team can help you decide what works best for you. The right treatment will make you more comfortable so you can get back to your normal routine. When your pain is under control, you will be better able to heal. Your pain will get better each day.

Tip

_____

As you wake up from surgery, tell your nurse if:

• *You need pain medicine.*

• *You feel sick to your stomach.*

• *Your legs or feet hurt, tingle or feel numb.*

Pain medicine

After surgery you will receive medicine for pain. For severe pain, you may receive strong medicines called narcotics. (Morphine, Dilaudid and codeine are examples of narcotics.) They work well, but they might make you drowsy, itchy or sick to your stomach. If you take narcotics, try to take the pills with food.

For mild or medium pain, you may be given drugs to reduce swelling and soreness (such as Tylenol, aspirin and ibuprofen). These may be used along with narcotics. They can have side effects, too, such as making you sick to your stomach.

There are different ways to take pain medicine. Depending on your doctor's orders, you may receive the medicine as a pill, as a shot or in your IV line.

After surgery, you may have a button you can push to control your pain yourself. This will pump pain medicine through your IV and into your body. The pump is set so you cannot give yourself too much medicine at one time. **Only you can touch this button. Family and other visitors may not touch this button.**

Here are some tips for taking pain medicine:

- Ask for medicine when you need it. Don't try to "tough it out"—this can make you feel worse. It's rare to get addicted to the kind of pain medicine used after surgery.

- Take your medicine as soon as you feel pain. Don't wait for pain to get worse before taking medicine.

- Medicine doesn't work the same for everyone. If yours isn't working, tell your nurse. He or she can try other medicines.

- Take pain medicine at least 45 minutes before physical therapy or other activities.

Your nurse will watch for side effects from the medicines. If you feel sick, "off" or uncomfortable after taking medicine, tell your nurse.

Keep in mind that medicine won't take away all of your pain. It helps to try other ways to relax and ease pain.

Tip

Tell your nurse if you feel sick after taking medicine, or if you just don't feel right. Your doctor may order a different medicine for you.

Ice, massage and movement

Ice packs, self-massage and moving your body into a different position all can help with pain. You may ask your nurse for ice or for a cold pack.

Relaxation

You can use your mind to reduce pain.

- **Visualize.** Imagine yourself in a nice place where you feel good. This might be at a beach, in a park or at home on your couch.

- **Distract yourself.** Do something to take your mind off the pain. For example, talk with a friend or play a game.

- **Listen to music.** For many people, calming music helps them feel better.

- **Breathe slowly.** If you focus on your breathing and let other thoughts go out of your mind, your pain may slip away for a while.

Visitors at the Hospital

During the first few days after surgery, you will be busy learning to use your new knee. You will need plenty of rest. Your care team will help you balance active times with rest periods.

The support of family and friends will help your recovery. But having too many visitors can take away from the rest you need. You may prefer to limit your visitors. Ask some people to save their visits until you are home.

Starting your recovery

Care equipment

Your care team may use special equipment to help you heal.

Continuous passive motion (CPM) machine: This machine gently bends and straightens your knee while you are lying in bed. This helps keep the joint moving and reduce swelling. If your doctor wants you to use the CPM machine, it will be adjusted to fit your knee. The amount your knee bends should increase regularly.

You may feel some discomfort at first. The machine will help speed your healing and keep your knee flexible, so it can bend as much as possible.

When using the machine, keep the center of your kneecap at the bend of the machine. Tell your nurse right away if you feel any change in your leg, such as numbness, burning or itching.

If you've had both knees replaced, you may have both legs in a CPM machine.

Knee immobilizer: Your doctor may have you wear a knee immobilizer. This is like a knee brace. It helps keep your leg straight and provides extra support for your knee when you walk. You will be shown how to wear it.

Breathing device (incentive spirometer): This helps you do your deep breathing exercises in the first few days after surgery.

Elastic stockings: These tight-fitting socks, known as TED stockings, may help prevent blood clots in your legs after surgery.

Tip

Do not get out of bed by yourself. Press the call button. A nurse will come help you.

Pillows

Do not put pillows under your knees at any time after knee surgery. This could cause problems with straightening your leg. Your nurse may place soft pillows or pads under your lower legs to keep your heels from getting sore.

Activity

At first you may not feel like doing anything at all, but movement and exercise are key to recovery. Soon you will begin doing exercises with the help of your physical therapist and nurses. But for now, remember:

- If you want to get out of bed, ask for help. Do not get out of bed by yourself.

- Some people have a sore back after surgery. Changing positions in bed once in a while will help.

Diet

Your diet may start with ice chips and liquids. You will begin eating regular meals as your body is able—when your stomach growls and you can pass gas. Tell your nurse if you'd like to meet with a dietician.

After your IV line is taken out, try to drink six to eight glasses of water each day. Drinking plenty of fluids helps prevent constipation (hard stools). Tell your nurse if you feel sick to your stomach and can't drink water.

Breathing exercises

Right after surgery, you will start your breathing exercises—deep breathing, coughing and using your breathing device. These help to keep your lungs clear and prevent problems like pneumonia.

Therapy

Therapy is very important to your recovery.

Tip

Take your pain medicine 45 minutes before therapy.

- **Physical therapy** focuses on range of motion in your knee—how far you can bend and straighten it. (Bending is called flexion. Straightening is called extension.) It teaches exercises to strengthen the muscles around your knee joint. It also teaches you how to walk and move safely with your new knee.

- **Occupational therapy** teaches you how to safely do everyday activities, such as bathing, getting dressed, cooking and cleaning. The therapist may suggest some equipment to make these tasks easier.

You will begin therapy soon after your surgery. You can start with ankle pumps and thigh squeezes while you're lying in bed. Do several of these exercises each hour while you're awake. You can also turn to your side in bed with help from a nurse.

The day after your operation, a nurse or physical therapist will help you stand up and sit in a chair. You may begin walking with help. You will learn how to safely move your knee and how to use a walker or crutches.

Each day of your hospital stay, you will do more exercises and walk a little more. You will work toward fully straightening and bending your knee. Over time, you will put more and more weight on your sore leg.

Before you leave the hospital, you will be given a set of exercises to do at home.

Tip

_____

Try to do things for yourself when you're in the hospital. This will help you heal faster.

Care plan

Your care plan describes what will happen while you are in the hospital. It helps you understand your treatment and the goals you and your health care team will work on before you go home. Your care plan may change depending on your needs. Feel free to ask questions of your care team during your hospital stay.

You will heal faster if you do as much as you can for yourself throughout your hospital stay. Your nurses will advise you on what you can do. Each day your physical activity should increase.

It's also important to express your feelings and concerns. Talk with your family or friends about what you might need after you leave the hospital.

Tip

Tell your nurse how you feel. He or she can give you medicine if you have pain or nausea (feel sick to your stomach).

Your goals

During your hospital stay, you'll work toward a number of goals with the help of your care team. Before you go home, you should be able to:

- Get safely in and out of bed, a chair and a car by yourself (or with a little help from your caregiver).

- Safely complete self-care activities, such as dressing and using the toilet. (You may use help or equipment as needed).

- Walk safely with a walker or crutches.

- Begin your home exercise program.

- Follow guidelines for knee safety.

- Know how to manage your pain.

- Know the signs of infection.

- Go to the toilet (urinate and move your bowels) as you did before your hospital stay.

- Eat a well-balanced diet to promote healing.

- Feel sure that you or your caregiver can meet your needs.

Each day of your hospital stay

- The nurse will check your blood pressure, pulse, temperature and breathing. He or she will also check the feeling, movement and color of your legs and feet. Your lungs and abdomen will be checked as well.

- If you feel pain or sick to your stomach, ask your nurse for medicine. He or she may ask you to rate your level of pain. Ask for pain medicine at least 45 minutes before doing any major activity or physical therapy.

- You may receive medicine to prevent blood clots. To make sure the medicine is working, you may be given blood tests.

- You will be urged to cough, take deep breaths and use your breathing device every 1 to 2 hours while you're awake.

- You will have physical therapy.

- You may have an ice pack on your knee to reduce pain and swelling.

- Your physical therapist will help you bend and straighten your knee. You may also use a continuous motion machine (CPM) to gently move your knee while you are in bed.

- Remember not to put a pillow under your knees.

- You may wear a knee immobilizer. (See page 35.)

- You'll wear elastic stockings to prevent blood clots in your legs. The stockings may be removed two to three times a day.

- Do ankle pumps 10 times an hour. (See page 21.) This improves blood flow in your legs.

First day after surgery

- Your nurse or therapist will help you stand up and sit in a chair. You may begin walking and exercising with help.

- You may begin pain pills.

- You may start eating regular foods.

- You may receive fluids, medicine and blood through an IV line in your arm.

- Your care team may remove your incision drain.

- Your nurse may change the bandage over the surgical area.

Second day after surgery

- You will walk and exercise at least two times with your physical therapist and nurses.

- You'll increase the bending of your knee.

- Your care team may remove your IV and bladder tubes. They may also remove your incision drain if they have not yet done so.

- Your nurse will change your bandages as needed.

- Talk with your nurse about your normal toilet habits. If you do not have a bowel movement today, you may need a laxative (medicine to help you go to the toilet).

- You will start occupational therapy.

Third day after surgery/Last day in the hospital

- Continue to increase your activity and knee bending.

- Make final plans for after your hospital stay. A social worker or care coordinator can help.

- Your physical therapist will teach you how to get in and out of a car and climb stairs. The therapist will also show you a home exercise program. Please bring this book to your physical therapy session.

- Ask a family member or your caregiver to come to a therapy session.

- Ask a family member to bring your walker or crutches to the hospital.

Tip

Bring this book with you to therapy sessions. It's a good idea to bring a family member or friend, too.

Getting ready to leave the hospital

Your care team will let you know when you can leave the hospital. Before you leave, your care team will review guidelines for:

- Knee safety

- Preventing falls

- Wound care

- Diet

- Problems to watch for

- Activity level

- Home exercises

- Equipment

- Bathing

- Elastic stockings

- Medicines

- Follow-up visits

These guidelines are covered in the next chapter. If you have any questions, ask your doctor or nurse.

Preventing Complications

Every surgery has its risks. With knee replacement surgery, the major risks include blood clots, infection, knee stiffness and loosening of the joint.

While you are in the hospital, your care team will take many steps to prevent these problems. For example:

- They will take your blood pressure, temperature and pulse often.

- They will check the movement, feeling, blood flow and pulse in your leg.

- You will do exercises that improve strength and blood flow.

- You will wear TED stockings (elastic socks) to help prevent blood clots.

- You will receive medicine to help keep blood clots from forming.

- You will do breathing exercises to keep your lungs clear and healthy.

- Your nurse will check your bandage and surgical wound often. Tubes will drain extra blood and fluid away from the wound area.

- You may use a CPM machine that slowly and gently moves your knee while you are in bed.

Some problems do not show up until long after surgery. Before you leave the hospital, you will learn what problems to watch for (see page 64).

Living with Your New Knee

By the time you leave the hospital, you should be able to do some things on your own, such as walk with crutches or a walker, get in and out of a bed or chair, and climb a few stairs.

Before you leave, you will be given advice and rules to follow. These rules help make your recovery safe and smooth. If you have any questions, be sure to ask your care team.

You will need someone to drive you home or to another care facility. Your doctor will let you know when you can start driving again after surgery.

What happens when you go home

Recovery takes time. Most people get back to their normal routine in three to six weeks. Many use a walker or crutches for three to four weeks, then use a cane for two or three more weeks. Most people can bend their knee to 90 degrees (a right angle) by the second week after surgery.

Full recovery can take two to three months, depending on your health and how well you do with therapy. If you had both knees replaced, it will take three months or longer to heal.

Medicines

At home, you'll keep taking the medicines your doctor prescribed. These may include drugs to prevent blood clots, such as Coumadin (warfarin) or aspirin. Another drug to prevent clots is heparin (Enoxaparin). This is taken as a shot. You or a family member will learn how to give a shot if you will take this medicine.

Your doctor will also prescribe pain pills. These can make therapy and knee exercises more comfortable. Take pain medicine 45 minutes before you exercise—it's easier to prevent pain than to treat it after it's started. Tell your nurse if you have trouble controlling pain. Most people stop needing pain medicine after a few weeks.

Some people also take medicine to help them sleep or to relax their muscles.

Wound care

You must keep the area around your incision (cut) clean while it heals. You will need someone to help you care for the wound.

- Look at it every day. Call your doctor if you see any redness, swelling or fluid draining from it, or if it feels warm or more painful.

- Change your bandage the way your care team showed you. Do not use any cream or ointment on the wound.

- If Steri-Strips (strips of tape) were used on the cut, they will fall off as it heals. You don't need to replace them.

- If staples were used, they will be removed at your next doctor visit or by a home health aide.

- If a clear suture (a stitch that looks like a fishing line) is sticking out from your incision, cut it flush with the skin. The rest of the suture will dissolve.

Knee immobilizer

If you cannot straighten your leg all the way, your doctor may ask you to keep wearing the knee immobilizer (knee brace) for a few weeks. Ask if you need to wear it at night.

Tip

Few people are pain-free when they leave the hospital. Expect to take pain killers for the first couple weeks.

Using ice on your knee

Ice can help reduce pain and swelling. It may be helpful to put an ice pack on your knee for about 15 minutes before and after you exercise. Pain and swelling can make it hard to move your knee.

Do not use a heating pad on your knee. This increases swelling in your knee joint.

Elastic socks

Keep wearing the white elastic stockings (TEDs) you got at the hospital. You should wear them until your first doctor visit after the surgery.

You can take the socks off twice a day for 15 minutes—ask someone to help you. It's fine to wash and dry them before you put them back on.

Massaging your knee

As your knee begins to heal, scar tissue will form between your skin and the bone. To make sure the scar tissue forms in a way that allows your knee to bend, you will need to massage (rub) the scar each day. Ask your doctor or physical therapist when you should start massaging the scar. Wait until the staples, sutures or Steri-Strips are removed.

To massage your scar:

1. While lying down or sitting in a chair, place your leg straight out in front of you. Keep your leg relaxed.

2. Put the palms of your hand gently on both sides of your scar.

3. Move your hands gently up and down and side to side. As you massage the scar, the skin should move over your bones.

Massage the scar gently and slowly for 30 to 60 seconds once or twice each day.

Therapy

You may still have physical therapy at the hospital or at home. Your care team will tell you how long you may need therapy.

The therapist will review your knee safety guidelines and help you with the exercises you'll do at home. You might also work on balance, safe walking and muscle strength. An occupational therapist may help you with day-to-day tasks.

Eating

When you leave the hospital, go back to your normal diet as soon as you can. Do not skip meals. Eat breakfast, lunch and dinner.

A well-balanced diet will help you feel good and recover quickly. Choose a range of fruits, vegetables, grains, milk products and meat. It's also important to drink plenty of fluids.

Be sure to include:

- **High-fiber foods.** Fiber helps keep your bowel movements regular and prevent constipation (hard stools). Good sources of fiber include whole grains, brown rice, cracked wheat (bulgur), oatmeal, popcorn, whole oats, rye and wheat. Fruits and vegetables are also great sources of fiber—plus they are low in fat and packed with nutrients.

- **High-calcium foods.** Calcium helps build strong bones. Good sources of calcium include milk, yogurt, cheese, enriched soymilk, tofu, soups made with milk, and dark green, leafy vegetables (such as kale or collard greens). Choose low-fat or fat-free dairy products. If you don't eat milk products, eat other foods that contain calcium. Ask your doctor if a calcium pill is a good idea for you.

- **Iron-rich foods.** This mineral helps your blood carry oxygen to every part of your body. Good sources of iron include lean meats, dark turkey meat, shellfish (such as shrimp), cooked dry beans or peas and whole grain breads.

If you have concerns about your eating plan, ask your nurse about setting up a visit with a dietician.

Tip

_____

Be sure to drink lots of water and other fluids. This will help prevent constipation (hard stools).

Bathing

Until your stitches or staples are removed, you will need to take sponge baths. Cover the stitches or staples with plastic to keep the wound dry when bathing.

You will be told when you can shower and get your wound wet. Use a tub or shower chair for support until you can get around more easily. (See page 58.) You will find tips on getting in and out of the tub on page 53.

Do not soak in a bathtub until your doctor says it's okay.

Preventing constipation

Many people have constipation (hard stools) after knee surgery. This is often caused by pain medicine, being less active and taking iron pills. To help prevent constipation:

- Drink eight to 10 glasses of fluid each day.

- Stay active.

- Eat more fiber. Choose whole grain breads, bran cereals and fresh fruits and vegetables.

- Stop using pain pills when you can.

If you have trouble with constipation, talk to your care team. They may suggest a stool softener, laxative or other medicine to relieve the problem.

Questions and Answers about Recovery

How long will I be in pain?

As your muscles and tissues heal, the pain you feel in your knee will get better. Most of the pain should go away in about a month. After that, it's normal to feel some aches once in a while, but severe pain is not normal.

When can I drive?

Your doctor will let you know when you can drive. Many surgeons advise against driving for at least four weeks after surgery. You need to be able to bend your knee far enough to sit in a car, and you need enough leg strength to operate the brake and accelerator. Do not drive while taking pain pills, because they can make your driving unsafe.

How soon can I take a bath or shower?

Your care team will let you know when you can take a shower or bath. You may have to wait several weeks before you can soak in the tub.

Will my new knee joint set off alarms at the airport?

Yes. When it does, tell the airport workers that you have an artificial knee. They will do a security check on you before you board the plane.

When can I have sex?

Ask your doctor. For most people, it's fine to have sex about four to six weeks after surgery. This allows time for the wound and muscles to heal. When you become sexually active again, use a firm mattress. Many people, men and women, find it easier to lie on their back during sex.

Movement and activity

After surgery, most people feel less pain than they have in a long time. You may find yourself able to do things you have avoided. Walking and other light activities will help you regain the use of your knee joint and muscles.

Still, you need to use your knee in safe ways until it heals. You also need to be careful when doing everyday tasks like getting out of bed, going up and down stairs, cooking and cleaning.

The following tips will help you do daily tasks without hurting your knee. As a general rule, avoid movements or positions that cause pain or discomfort in your knee.

Getting in and out of bed

To get into bed:

- Back up toward the bed until you feel it against your legs. Place your operated leg forward.

- Reaching back with one hand at a time, slowly lower yourself onto the edge of the bed.

- Scoot back until your thighs are supported by the edge of the bed.

- Support your upper body with your arms, then bring your legs into the bed. To lift your operated leg, you may need to use a crutch, cane, belt or leg lifter (see page 56). Or ask someone for help.

Tip
_____

You may lie on your side when you're in bed. Do not put a pillow under your knee while lying on your back.

To get out of bed:

- Come to a sitting position in the bed.

- Turn your body and move your legs off the bed. To move your leg, you may need to use a crutch, cane, belt or leg lifter (see page 56). Or ask someone for help.

- Keep your body in a straight line with your legs. Move to sit at the edge of the bed.

- Place your operated leg forward.

- Push off the bed and stand up.

Keep your body and legs in a straight line. You will need to bend your "good" knee when getting out of bed.

Using a walker or crutches

Use a walker or crutches until your care team tells you to stop. Your doctor will let you know how much weight you can place on your leg.

To walk:

- Stand up straight, with your weight evenly balanced on the walker or crutches. Keep the walker flat on the floor.

- Move the walker or crutches forward a little. Then, step forward. Lift your operated leg so that the heel of your foot touches the floor first.

- Try to walk as smoothly as you can. Over time you will put more and more weight on your leg.

- Do not twist or pivot on your operated leg. Take small steps and turn toward your strong leg.

From Walker to Cane

Many people use a walker for the first several weeks after knee surgery. A walker helps with balance and keeps you from falling. After that, you may use a cane for several more weeks until you get your strength and balance back.

You are ready to use a cane when:

- You can stand and balance without your walker.

- Your weight is placed fully on both feet.

- You no longer lean on your hands when using your walker.

Carry your cane or crutch in the hand opposite your sore leg. For example, if you had surgery on your left knee, use the cane with your right hand.

To sit:

- Back up until you feel the chair against the back of your legs.

- Slide your operated leg forward, then lower yourself slowly into the chair. Use the armrests.

To stand:

- Come to the edge of the chair with your operated leg out in front of you.

- Use both arms to push yourself up to standing, then reach for your walker.

- Do not use the walker to pull yourself up.

Tip

Never use your walker to pull yourself up from a seated position.

Getting on and off an armless chair

To sit:

- Approach the chair from the side.

- Slide your operated leg in front of you.

- Holding the edge of the seat and the back of the chair, slowly sit down. Then, turn to face forward in the chair.

To stand:

- Turn your body so you are sitting sideways in the chair.

- Slide your operated leg in front of you.

- Push up from the chair with both hands. Place one hand on the back of the chair.

- When your balance is steady, reach for your walker or crutches.

Using the toilet

You may need to use a toilet with a raised seat. (See page 56.)

- To sit down, back up to the toilet until you can feel it against your legs.

- Move your operated leg forward. Reach back with both hands and grab the safety rails, armrests or raised toilet seat.

- Slowly lower yourself onto the toilet, using both arms.

- To stand up, slide to the edge of the toilet and move your operated leg forward. Place both hands behind you on the toilet seat.

- Push off with both arms to raise yourself off the toilet.

- When your balance is steady, reach for your walker or crutches. Never try to pull yourself up from the toilet by grabbing your walker.

Tip

_____

Do not sit for more than one hour at a time. (This includes riding in a car.) Get up and stretch or walk a little. Change your position (sitting, walking, lying flat) every hour while you're awake.

Bathing

When you start taking baths and showers, it's a good idea to have handrails or grab bars in the tub. These will help with balance and support. You can also use a long-handled sponge and a hand-held showerhead.

If you use a bathtub, you will sit on a tub chair with your leg straight. (See page 58.) The heel should rest on the edge of the tub.

Your occupational therapist can give you tips to make bathing easier. The first few times you take a bath or shower, have someone nearby in case you need help.

To bathe or shower:

- Use a tub chair in the bathtub or shower. Do not sit on the floor of the bathtub.

- Come up to the bathtub so that the tub chair is at your side. Place your operated leg forward.

- Reach with one hand to the back of the tub seat or handrail. Reach the other hand to the front edge of the tub seat. Then, slowly turn and sit. Keep both hands on the tub seat or handrail while you lower yourself.

- Lift one leg into the tub at a time. Use a cane, crutch, belt or leg lifter to lift your operated leg. Or ask someone to help you.

- To get out of the tub, use a cane, crutch or belt to lift your operated leg.

- Push up from the chair with both hands, or use the handrails to pull yourself up.

- When your balance is steady, reach for your walker or crutches.

Use a tub chair to get in or out of the bathtub or shower.

When bathing, sit on your tub chair with your heel resting on the tub's edge. A hand-held showerhead makes bathing easier.

Reaching, bending and carrying

You will need some help with laundry, cleaning and shopping when you get home. When you start doing housework, follow these tips:

Tip

_____

Use equipment—a long-handled reacher, a walker basket, a rolling cart—to make your tasks easier.

- Use a long-handled reacher to turn on lights or grab things that are beyond arm's length. (See page 56.) Do not bend to reach in low cupboards.

- Do not carry or hold things in your hands while using a walker or crutches. Instead, carry things in an apron, pocket, fanny pack, backpack or walker basket.

- Do not reach too far when sliding items across a counter.

- Do not stand on tiptoes or chairs to reach high cupboards or storage areas.

- Use a rolling cart to carry hot, heavy or fragile items.

- Use a high stool (without wheels) when you cook or do dishes.

Going up and down stairs

- Remember: "Up with the good" and "down with the bad." Go up the step with your good leg first. Then bring your other leg up to the same step. Go down with your "bad" leg first. Then bring your good leg down to the same step.

- Use the handrails for support.

- Do not try to climb steps that are higher than the standard height (7 inches).

Getting in and out of a car

Move your car seat back as far as it goes to increase the legroom. When you are getting in or out of the car, have the driver park away from the curb and not on a hill.

To get into a car:

- Back up to the front seat until you feel it at the back of your legs. Slide your operated leg forward.

- Reach back and find a stable place to hold on to, such as the dashboard and back of the seat. Slowly lower yourself onto the seat without twisting your body.

- Scoot back onto the seat. Keeping your body in line with your legs, slowly turn your body and lift your legs into the car so you are facing forward. Ask someone to help you lift your operated leg, or use a cane or crutch to lift it yourself.

- A plastic bag on the car seat may help you move more easily.

To get out of a car:

- Slowly turn your body as you move your legs out of the car. Keep your body in line with your legs. Use a cane or crutch to lift your operated leg, or ask someone else to do it.

- Scoot to the edge of the seat and put your feet on the street (not the curb).

- Push with your arms and use your good leg to stand.

- When your balance is steady, reach for your walker or crutches.

Equipment that can help

You can buy or rent special equipment to make tasks easier. You will need to use a walking aid—a walker, crutches or a cane. Your health care team may also want you to use a leg lifter, a raised toilet seat and a reacher. You may need other items as well.

The occupational therapist will show you how to get and use your equipment before you leave the hospital. (See "Where to get health equipment," page 59, and Resources, pages 67 and 68.)

Health insurance may cover only the cost of a walking aid. Call your insurance company to find out if anything else is covered.

Walking aids

A walker, crutches or a cane will help you walk after surgery.

Raised toilet seat

This makes it easier for you to get on and off the toilet.

Commode

A portable toilet allows you to stay on one floor of your home if you don't have a bathroom on each level.

Reacher

A reacher helps you grab things that are too high or low. It can also help you put clothes on.

Leg lifter

Use a leg lifter to move your operated leg safely in and out of a bed, car or bathtub.

Long-handled sponge

Use this to wash your feet, legs and back without bending.

Hand-held showerhead

This lets you control the spray of water while sitting down in a tub or shower.

Elastic laces

Elastic laces allow you to put on shoes that are already tied.

Long-handled shoehorn

With the shoehorn, you can put your foot into a shoe without bending.

Sock aid

A sock aid helps you put on socks without bending.

Grab bars

Install grab bars to hold onto when getting on or off the toilet and in or out of the tub or shower.

Toilet tongs

Tongs allow you to use toilet paper without twisting your body.

Dressing stick

You can use a dressing stick to get dressed without bending. To remove socks, slide the dressing stick down into the sock, by the heel. Push the sock off. To put on pants:

1. Hook the stick in the pants' belt loop at the front of the leg you are dressing first, near the zipper.

2. Lower the pants to the floor and put your foot in.

3. Use the stick to pull the pants up to where you can reach them with your hand.

4. Repeat with the other leg.

Tub or shower chair

This is useful if you can't stand up long enough to shower, or if you have trouble getting in or out of the tub. It is often used with a hand-held showerhead.

Tub transfer bench

A bench keeps you from stepping over the edge of the bathtub. It is useful for people who cannot bear full weight on their leg (who have a "weight-bearing restriction"). To use the bench:

1. Come to the edge of the tub and turn around so you feel the bench at the back of your knees.

2. Lower yourself onto the bench and turn toward the tub.

3. Lift your feet over the edge of the tub one at a time while keeping your leg straight.

4. To get out of the tub, use the same process in reverse.

Clamp-on tub rail

You can hold onto this when getting in and out of the bathtub. This must be installed on the edge of your tub.

Where to Get Health Care Equipment

To find the items you need, try these ideas:

- Borrow them from friends or family.

- Call your local American Legion, VFW or Lions Club. They often have health care equipment that you can borrow.

- Call your local drugstore to see what items the store carries.

- Your care team may have mail-order catalogs that sell a range of equipment.

- Look in the Yellow Pages under "disabled persons' assistance" or "home health services" for agencies that sell equipment.

Work and hobbies

Ask your doctor when you can go back to work. If you have a desk job, you may be able to return to work fairly soon. It may take longer to go back to jobs that involve driving, walking or standing.

Three to six weeks after surgery, you should be able to do simple activities such as shopping and light housework. Many hobbies are fine to do soon after surgery. They are a good way to pass the time as you're recovering. But if your hobby involves heavy lifting or activity, hold off. Talk to your doctor if you are unsure about your activity level.

Exercise

Exercise can help prevent problems after surgery. It also builds your strength so you can get back to your normal routine.

Your leg muscles probably feel weak because you did not use them much when your knee was giving you trouble. After the surgery, regular exercise will help strengthen your weak muscles. The knee exercises you learned will make your knee stronger, allowing it to move smoothly and without pain.

Exercise also helps prevent constipation (hard stools). It keeps your joints flexible (able to move easily), improves muscle tone and makes you feel good. Without it, you will be weak and stiff.

Knee exercises

Your physical therapist will show you what exercises to do at home and how to do them correctly. Do these exercises two times a day for at least three months.

Most exercises can be done lying down. Your bed is a good place. Don't lie on the floor.

It's normal to feel a little sore after exercise. But if you feel a lot of pain or muscle aches, talk to your care team.

Knee Exercises to Do at Home

Keep doing the exercises you practiced before surgery. But now that your home, you should add these exercises to your daily routine.

Knee bends

Sit on a chair with your feet on the floor. Pull your leg back toward the chair as much as you can. You will feel the stretch in your knee. Hold the stretch for 10 to 15 seconds. Return to the starting position and relax. Repeat 10 times. Do this two times a day for three months.

Work up to holding the stretch for 30 seconds. The longer you hold it, the better the stretch. To increase the stretch, scoot forward on the chair.

Knee straightening

Sit in a sturdy chair. Rest the heel of your operated leg on another chair or on a footstool in front of you. Or you can lie in bed with a pillow under your ankle or heel. You should feel a stretch at the back of your knee. Work on straightening your knee for 10 to 15 minutes. Do this two times a day for three months.

Knee swings

Sit on the edge of a bed so that your feet do not touch the floor. Allow your knees to bend. Swing your operated leg back and forth gently. Keep swinging it for two to three minutes. Do this two times a day for three months.

Walking

Besides your home exercise program, make time each day for walking. Walking is a good form of physical therapy and makes your leg muscles stronger. It also builds your endurance. This means you'll be able to do more without feeling as tired.

Start by walking around your home at least four times each day. Trips to the bathroom or kitchen are not enough. Keep using your walker or crutches until your doctor tells you to stop. Later you can use a cane until you are steady enough to walk without one.

Work your way up to walking outdoors. At first, walk for 5 to 10 minutes a few times a day. As you become stronger, you may be able to walk for 20 to 30 minutes. After you have fully recovered, regular walks will help keep you strong.

Staying active

Some sports, such as basketball and running, are not good choices after knee replacement. But over time, most people are able to enjoy lighter activities, including golf, dancing and riding a bike.

Good choices for staying active include:

- Swimming

- Walking

- Water aerobics

- Riding a bike or stationary cycle

- Golf

- Dancing

- Cross-country skiing

These help you stay fit without too much wear on your new joint. But some activities will increase the risk of problems.

Avoid these unless you have your doctor's approval:

- Jogging and running

- High-impact exercise, such as aerobics

- Tennis

- Jumping sports, such as basketball

- Racquetball

- Contact sports, such as football

- Downhill skiing

- Hard hiking

Follow-up visits

Your first follow-up visit to your doctor will be four to six weeks after you leave the hospital. (You may come back sooner to have your staples taken out.) At this time, the doctor will do a physical exam and make sure the wound is healing well. You may also have X-rays taken of your knee.

You will have more follow-up visits during the year to see how well you are doing. After the first year, most people can see their doctor once a year.

Preventing problems

After knee surgery, you need to watch for infections and other problems. Some of these problems could happen soon after surgery, while others might not show up until months or even years later.

Symptoms to watch for

Call your doctor right away if:

- Your leg is cool to the touch or a gray color.

- You feel numbness or tingling in your leg.

- You get a temperature of 101°F (38°C) or higher.

- You have chills.

- The area around the wound becomes more swollen, warm, red or painful.

- Fluid, pus or bright red blood comes out of the incision.

- You have increasing pain that is not helped by medicine, rest or ice packs.

- You have sudden, severe knee pain.

- You notice new or sudden swelling or pain in your thigh or calf.

- There is a burning feeling or foul odor when you urinate (pass water when going to the toilet), or you feel like you have to go more often than usual.

- You can't put weight on your leg (and you could before).

- You fall.

Preventing infection

If you get an infection caused by germs anywhere in your body, the germs could travel to your new knee. Though rare, an infection in your knee joint is a serious problem. The germs can settle around the new joint, and this may be hard to treat. Infection usually means you need more surgery.

To prevent infection, you need to be extra careful from now on. If you get an illness, such as strep throat or pneumonia, tell your doctor right away. He or she will give you antibiotic medicine to stop the germs from spreading.

You will need to tell other care providers that you have had a joint replaced. This is true if you will have dental work or any type of surgery or procedure that may expose you to germs. You will need to take antibiotic medicine before having dental work or another procedure.

You will receive a medical alert card to carry in your wallet or billfold. In an emergency, this will tell care providers that you have an artificial knee.

Since an infection can develop in your knee joint many years after surgery, you will need to follow these rules all the time.

Tip

From now on, you must take antibiotic medicine before having any dental work or medical procedure.

The key to recovery

Your doctors, nurses, therapists and other members of your care team want to do everything possible to give you a pain-free, working knee. But remember, you play a key role in the success of your knee replacement. You can increase the odds of a smooth recovery by having a positive attitude, doing your exercises every day, following your knee safety rules and watching for problems.

As the days go by, you will feel stronger, move more easily and have more energy. Then you can enjoy your new knee and the freedom it brings.

Resources

American Academy of Orthopaedic Surgeons
6300 North River Road
Rosemount, Illinois 60018
Phone: 847-823-7186 or 800-824-AAOS [2267]
www.aaos.org
    The academy provides education and services for surgeons who treat disorders of the bones, joints, ligaments, muscles and tendons. It also provides information for patients.

American Association of Hip and Knee Surgeons
6300 North River Road, Suite 615
Rosemount, Illinois 60018
Phone: 847-698-1200
www.aahks.org/index.asp/fuseaction/patients.main
    The AAHKS provides information and education to surgeons as well as patients having hip or knee surgery. Also offers information on minimally invasive surgery.

American Physical Therapy Association
1111 North Fairfax Street
Alexandria, Virginia 22314
Phone: 703-684-2782 or 800-999-2782
www.apta.org
    This national organization for physical therapists seeks to improve research, public understanding and education about physical therapy.

Arthritis Foundation
P.O. Box 7669
Atlanta, Georgia 30357
Phone: 404-872-7100
www.arthritis.org
    The foundation publishes pamphlets and other information for people who have arthritis.

Fairview Health Services
www.fairview.org

National Institute of Arthritis and Musculoskeletal and Skin Diseases Information Clearinghouse
NIAMS/National Institutes of Health
1 AMS Circle
Bethesda, Maryland 20892
Phone: 301-495-4484 or 877-22-NIAMS [226-4267]
TTY: 301-565-2966
www.niams.nih.gov

The clearinghouse provides information about various forms of arthritis and bone, muscle and skin diseases.

University of Minnesota Department of Orthopaedics
www.ortho.umn.edu/ortho/academic/divisions/adult_reconstruction/patients.html

Includes frequently asked questions about hip and knee replacement.

Glossary

acute pain: intense, severe pain that comes on suddenly

analgesic: pain medicine

anesthesia: medicine to remove sensation from all of the body (general anesthesia) or part of it (local anesthesia)

antibiotics: drugs that kill or stop the growth of bacteria (germs)

anti-inflammatories: drugs that reduce pain and swelling

arthritis: pain, swelling and stiffness in the joints

assistive device: walker, dressing stick, raised toilet or other item to help you do daily activities

cartilage: white or yellow tissue that connects parts of the body

catheter: a flexible tube that is put into the body to bring in or take out fluids

cement: a product used to attach the artificial joint to your bone, working like cement between the bricks of a wall

chronic pain: mild to severe pain that lasts a long time, usually more than two or three months

continuous passive motion (CPM) machine: device that slowly moves your knee back and forth to exercise your new joint after surgery

deep vein thrombosis (DVT): blood clots in the calf or thigh

extension: straightening of a joint

femur: thighbone

flexion: bending of a joint

flexion limit: how much you can bend your knee

Hemovac: machine that collects the fluid from your wound after surgery

immobilizer: brace that provides support for the knee

incentive spirometer: machine that helps you breathe deeply so you can exercise your lungs and keep them clear

incision: surgical cut or wound

infection: invasion of the body by harmful germs; common symptoms include pain, swelling and red, warm skin

IV (intravenous) tube: a tube for putting fluids into a vein

loosening: when the artificial joint becomes detached or wears away from the bone

operated leg: the leg that you had surgery on

orthopedic surgeon: a surgeon who treats disorders of the bones and joints

osteoarthritis: "wear and tear" arthritis, marked by the wearing away of cartilage in the joint

OT: occupational therapy; provides help with daily activities such as dressing, using the toilet, bathing and household tasks

patella: kneecap; the bone at the front of the knee joint that you feel when you touch your knee

PCA pump: patient-controlled analgesia pump; a machine that gives pain medicine, which you control with a button

prosthesis: artificial joint

PT: physical therapy; helps with exercises and your ability to move and walk

rehabilitation (rehab): physical and occupational therapy

sutures: surgical stitches

TEDs: white elastic socks used to prevent blood clots

tibia: shinbone

weight-bearing status: how much weight you can put on your operated leg

Bibliography

Allina Health System. *Total Hip Replacement.* First edition. Minneapolis: Allina Press, 2004.

Allina Health System. *Total Knee Replacement.* First edition. Minneapolis: Allina Press, 2004.

American Academy of Orthopaedic Surgeons. Surgical Treatment of Osteoarthritis of the Knee. July 2003. At: http://www.orthoinfo.aaos.org/fact/thr_report.cfm?Thread_ID=442&topcategory=Arthritis.

American Academy of Orthopaedic Surgeons. Total Hip Replacement Exercise Guide. 2000. At: http://www.orthoinfo.aaos.org/booklet/view_report.cfm?Thread_ID=20&topcategory=Hip.

Fairview Health Services. *Before Your Surgery.* Minneapolis: Fairview Press, 2004.

———. "Fairview-University Medical Center Orthopaedic Clinic." 2004. At: http://www.fairview.org/provider/clinicbio.asp?BID=561. Accessed January 18, 2005.

———. *You and Your Total Knee Replacement.* Minneapolis: Fairview Health Services, 1997.

Grelsamer, Ronald P. *What Your Doctor May Not Tell You about Hip and Knee Replacement Surgery: Everything You Need to Know to Make the Right Decisions.* New York: Warner Books, 2004.

Healthpages.org. "A Patient's Guide to Total Knee Replacement Surgery." May 17, 1997. At: http://www.healthpages.org/AHP/LIBRARY/HLTHTOP/TKR/. Accessed April 13, 2005.

Mayo Clinic. "Total Hip Replacement: Relieve Pain, Improve Mobility." April 18, 2003. At: http://www.mayoclinic.com/invoke.cfm?id=9BE7ADB-2D2C-478908D784568379C6B70.

Mayo Clinic. "Knee Replacement Surgery at Mayo Clinic in Jacksonville, 2004." At: http://www.mayoclinic.org/kneereplacement-jax/. Accessed October 22, 2004.

Mayo Clinic. "Total Knee Replacement". Mc2111. October 2002.

MayoClinic.com, "Advance Directives: Make Your Medical Care Wishes Known." July 16, 2003. At: http://www.mayoclinic.com/invoke.cfm?id=HA00014. Accessed January 25, 2005.

———. "Knee Pain." September 22, 2004. At: http://www.http://www. mayoclinic.com/invoke.cfm?objectid=DS0555. Accessed April 13, 2005.

———. "Knee Replacement: Surgery Can Relieve Pain." June 17, 2004. At: http://www.http://www.mayoclinic.com/invoke. cfm?objectid=HQ00977. Accessed April 13, 2005.

Trahair, Richard. *All about Hip Replacement: A Patient's Guide.* Melbourne: Oxford University Press, 2000.

University of Virginia Health System. "Total Hip Replacement." November 19, 2002. At: http://www.healthsystem.virginia.edu:80/internet/ orthopaedics/thr.cfm. Accessed July 20, 2004.

University of Washington Department of Orthopaedics and Sports Medicine. "Total Knee Replacement: A Patient's Guide." N.d. At: http:// www.orthop.washington.edu/faculty/Leopold/totalknee/print. Accessed October 22, 2004.

Virtual Hospital, University of Iowa Department of Orthopaedics. "Total Knee Replacement: A Patient Guide." June 2004. At: http://www. vh.org/adult/patient/orthopaedics/kneereplacement/. Accessed April 13, 2005.